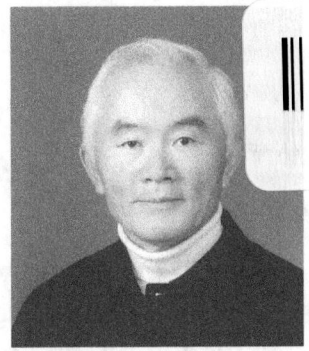

Tong Kim, a poet and painter, was born in Tong Young, South Korea in 1943. He worked as a barber in a mountain-side village on weekends to pay for his high school tuition and graduated with a MBA degree from Yonsei University in Seoul.

He worked as a bank assistant manager, but quit and moved to southern California in 1973 with hopes of retirement within 15 years. He began his career as a kitchen assistant working 16 hours a day, frugally saving enough to start a gas station and grocery store business. He survived 3 armed robberies. That led to the hotel business from which he was able to comfortably retire from in 1980.

Living in Monterey, he served as chairman of the Korean American Association and Korean Language School.

Between 1982 and 1999, his overwhelming curiosity and desire (religion, god, various studies and activities) led him to spend most of his time in South Korea searching for the meaning of life.

In 1989, after being fascinated by Monet's Water Lily, he wondered what would be the Asian version of the Water Lily. This inspired him to start painting. Considering the canvas as a fiancee, he refuses to use a knife on it. After two years of painting, more than half of his first private exhibition contained paintings with the water lily theme.

He also held additional exhibitions: three times in South Korea, two times in Japan, and once in the United States.

In 1999, he published "Stopped watch", a collection of poems and essays.

In the late summer of that same year, he set up a tent to live in for his 100 days of camping in the mountains. He ate twice a day, meditated, and gazed at the same sun that rose morning after morning. While the sun was still sleeping in the morning, he cooked a warm meal for the mountain rat family and came down from the mountain.

In 2005, he won awards at the public competition held by the Contemporary Poetry publisher, in South Korea. He submitted "The Horizon" and four other poems. "The Horizon" took him three years to perfect.

In 2008, he published "Tomorrow Today," a collection of poems and essays.

In 2013, he published "609020" in Korean.

In 2014, he published "609020" (Rainbow Ssambap)

in English.

Author:

Tong P. Kim

tongpkim@gmail.com

Publisher:

Carmel Valley Lodge

8 Ford Rd, Carmel Valley
California, 93924

(831)659-2261

www.valleylodge.com

Special thanks to Peter Krasa and Moon Choe

Author's Note I

The enlightenment and wisdom have time.

If it is not the time

You can't see, hear, and accept it.

Whatever you do

Whatever you choose

All that you do is your share

Any idea

No matter what the behavior

This all

This is because the share of the self.

"60 90 20"

Let you meet the moment

Let you know the moment

Let you earn time.

Author's Note II

I attended a speech by a very famous religious leader. I expected to hear great wisdom from him, but I only heard, basically, to be nice to another human being. Who doesn't know that! Everybody knows that. Why does he have such fame and respect? Later I realized that his greatness is his life's dedication to it; reminding people again and again how being nice to one another is important for humanity.

I am neither a doctor nor a nutritionist; I just might have a little more knowledge than the average person regarding the relationship between what we eat and the diseases we contract. Most of the information and knowledge in this book can easily be found in books and on the Internet. I just want to remind you through this book that right eating brings health and happiness in your life and all of our lives. I am happy to share my experiences and knowledge with others and to remind them repeatedly what we should eat.

Contents

Chapter I: Rainbow Ssambap®

Chapter II: Thoughts

Chapter III: Diseases

Chapter IV: Food is Everything

Chapter V: Nothing New, Looks Novel

Chapter I

Rainbow Ssambap®

How It Started

It is very difficult to discontinue eating food that we have eaten our whole lives, even if we know that the food isn't good for our body. Changing our eating habits from our parents' within a short period is a monumental task.

I have suffered from a digestive problem since I was a child. I couldn't even digest a single bowl of cooked rice while other kids could eat three bowls of rice per day. I was the thinnest student at school. I decided to improve my health when I was twenty-years old. I started avoiding salty, spicy, processed, and fast foods, and stopped drinking coffee, tea, and soft drinks. Soon my digestive system got better.

I stopped eating meat and dairy products in my early 40's. I became a dedicated vegetarian after I stopped eating fish when I was in my 60's; since then, I eat like the herbivores that live in the wild. My vegetarian diet has changed many times through my experiments with vegetables. Rainbow Ssambap® is the product of many years of my experiments and trials.

I have eaten three meals a day with Rainbow Ssambap® for many years and it has improved my health and stamina. I was surprised by the level of improvement. My wife asked me to have a comprehensive medical examination; if the result is good then she promised me that she would eat Rainbow Ssambap® every day, as I have been. For the first time in my life, I took a comprehensive medical exam in the fall of 2012. The result was very good; the doctor told me that my physical age was around 30 years old, 40 years younger than my actual age. The doctor asked me what the secret was. I gave credit to Rainbow Ssambap®.

I know that Rainbow Ssambap® has been great for my health, but there wasn't proof of the effectiveness of it. After my examination, I realized that it is great and that I should share it with other people, so they can have healthier and happier lives.

I realized my mission for the rest of my life was to share Rainbow Ssambap®. Since then I have been promoting Rainbow Ssambap® religiously. Some of my friends jokingly call me a "Rainbow Ssambap® cult leader." I don't mind since I am spreading a wonderful thing, not a strange belief.

Don't you want to join the Rainbow Ssambap® cult to spread this wonderful vegetarian dish to the world, to protect humankind from all of the commercialized foods, and make healthier and peaceful humanity?

Some say

It was born from the Heaven and the Ocean

Some mention

That it occasionally builds a double rainbow

bridge

Some claim

A cloud was doing a dangerous tightrope

walking

Others say

It is a cliff of a thousand miles fall

Poem -Horizon-

How to Make Rainbow Ssambap®

Please check "How to make Rainbow Ssambap®" video at www.youtube.com by typing Rainbow Ssambap®.

A Review by **Michelle Wen** on YouTube.

"This is amazing green salad! I'm surprised with the result; I feel much higher energy level than before, skin looks much brighter, I lost weight in a healthy way. My girlfriends are trying this now, thanks!"

You need nuts (almonds, cashews, walnuts), fresh vegetables (one beet, three tomatoes, 20 cherry tomatoes, one carrot, and any other vegetable that you want to eat), and fruits (apples, blueberries, bananas, lemons, avocados, etc.), but not salt, water, and food additives.

1) Make a base - Put five sliced tomatoes at the bottom of the blender, and put one sliced beet, one carrot, two bananas, one avocado, 20 almonds, 20 cashews, and five walnuts on top of it and blend them all together.

2) Pour it into a large bowl up to 1/3 of the bowl.

3) Add blueberries, strawberries, cherry tomatoes, one chopped apple, ½ of a lemon, some lettuce, and any other vegetables, nuts, or fruits that you want to eat.

4) Mix and eat it.

Please never put salt or food additives.

One of the good aspects of the Rainbow Ssambap® is that you can prepare it a few days in advance. If you make enough Rainbow Ssambap® base, (step one), for two days and save it in the refrigerator, you can later add step 3 and enjoy. It is faster and more convenient than cooking Ramen or soup.

With a bowl of water

Hand full of light

on land

in heaven

Rainbow Ssambap

Overflow of joy

Overflow of energy

Arise double rainbows

for heaven

-Poem: Rainbow Ssambap

Revolution in the Kitchen by the Rainbow Ssambap®

Once you adapt Rainbow Ssambap® as your main food, you will soon realize that you don't need all the fancy kitchen equipment. You only need a few nice bowls, a knife, a cutting board, spoons, a refrigerator, containers for Rainbow Ssambap® ingredients, and a blender. You don't even need a dishwasher; it is very easy to clean dishes after eating Rainbow Ssambap® since it doesn't have oily or sticky stuff on it. You simply need to rinse it with water. You don't need a cooktop range or oven as they destroy many nutrients and enzymes in our food.

Another convenient aspect of the Rainbow Ssambap® is that anyone can make it. You don't have to be the best chef! Anyone who is big enough to make it can create it since it doesn't require special technique or know how. So it finally gives people more time outside of the kitchen.

You will no longer see meat, fish, milk and other dairy products, fast foods, and any seasoning or sauces in the refrigerator, but in their place- fruits, vegetables, beans, nuts, and seeds. Even your refrigerator looks and feels healthier.

Temptation of Unhealthy Food That You Ate

I have been a vegetarian for a long time so I didn't have any problem eating Rainbow Ssambap® however some people who have tried it have had cravings for old food that they used to eat. It is not as severe as drug withdrawal but they complained about great cravings for oily food or meat for the first few weeks. I have not found supporting medical documentation; however, I believe the shrunken fat cells send chemical signals to the brain to supply fat to cells so it can fully store fat. I hope you understand the importance of this diet before you start eating Rainbow Ssambap® so you can overcome the cravings and successfully become a vegetarian. I don't want you to fail because you give in to the craving.

> What I was
>
> Winding up the path
>
> Unwinding down the path
>
> Rolling on the path
>
> Asingle wheel
>
> A single wagon
>
> That, I was.
>
> -Poem: Training for life

Change of Taste and Smell

After successfully eating Rainbow Ssambap® for a few months, many people have told me that their preference for tastes and smells has changed. Foods people used to enjoy, such as ice cream, chocolate, cake, and steak, no longer tasted good. They were surprised by these changes. They also told me that they no longer like the smells that they used to like, such as the smell of a BBQ. I think it's a clear result of eating Rainbow Ssambap®. After we experience nature-made foods that are in their raw state, we realize how we were fooled by the commercialized and/or cooked foods, and through consumption, which has hurt our health, our taste and smell preferences have changed.

Rainbow Ssambap® and Enzymes

An enzyme is a protein molecule that catalyzes or speeds up a biological reaction. It can be used repeatedly as a catalyst. Enzymes, which are simply a biological catalyst, control cellular metabolism by controlling the rate of production of new products. The chemical changes that constitute biological processes in all living things require catalysts to trigger them. Our lifespan is governed by our enzyme supply and enzymes in foods increase our enzyme potential. When the enzyme content in our body becomes so low that our metabolism cannot continue, we then die. Raw fruits and vegetables are high in enzymes and Rainbow Ssambap® has plenty of enzymes since it is uncooked raw fruits, nuts, beans and vegetables.

-Eat Like a Deer

No Cancer

-Eat Like a Rabbit

Stop High Blood Pressure

Prevent Heart Disease.

-Eat Like a Cow

No More Fear and Anxiety

-Laugh and Rejoice

HAPPINESS

Poem -Vegan-

Cooking Kills Enzymes and People

If we cook raw food higher than 118 degrees (48 degrees Celsius), it will destroy the enzymes. Animals that live exclusively on a raw food diet don't develop degenerative diseases such as cancer, diabetes, and heart diseases because of the abundance of enzymes present. When they were fed cooked food in captivity, they developed these degenerative diseases. When they were fed with raw food again, their health improved. We have degenerative diseases mainly due to eating cooked foods that have damaged enzymes. In order to avoid these diseases, we should eat raw foods, fruits, nuts, beans and vegetables.

Chapter II

Thoughts
How Long Should Humans Live?

According to Science, the life of all animals, including humans, is 6 to 7 times of their growth period. The growth period of humans ends between 22- and 24-years-old. Therefore, theoretically, humans should live between 132 and 168 years with happiness and health. Unfortunately, most people only live half of that given life.

The reasons are as follows:

- Eating cooked food.
- Don't want to change eating habits inherited from parents.
- People are born with digestive organs meant for raw vegetables, fruits, beans, and nuts, but not meat.
- Eating too much salt and food additives. Not all natural foods require salt or spices.
- Peoples' reliance on medicine, health supplements, and doctors.
- People increasingly eat processed food and instant food, and consume soft drinks.

What Do We Eat?

Americans get about 42 percent of their calories from meat that has no fiber, vitamec or phytochemicals which detoxifies our body, and 52 percent from carbohydrates, processed and refined oil, and only five percent from vegetables, fruits, beans, and nuts. Easy fast food and processed convenience foods are prevalent in the American diet.

In Bed

Ask your digestive organs about your diet today while massaging your stomach in bed, "Organs, have you been happy today?" The question would be answered in the morning at the toilet. If it is happy, it will give an easy bowl movement. Your organs will abandon you if you eat bad food and take medicines that do not harmonize with your body. You could potentially get a serious illness and it would be extremely painful and restricting. When you eat the right foods, maintain a positive state of mind, and take care of your body, you will be saved from negative consequences. The importance of your organs is irreplaceable. Organs are not accessories of the body, but have conscious and independent personalities.

Know It After It Has Changed

You will know the flavor and taste of the season after the season matures. When there is the scent of spring flowers in the air, we know that spring is here. In the arms of the warm spring, we forget the high and cold winds. We realize and are shocked about how we lived after getting a serious illness and being on an operating table. We don't know what to do in front of the harsh winter cold wind. Spring is a privilege given to those who are ready. Rainbow Ssambap® is the spring; we know it when we are in the arms of spring. We know that whether cooked food, meat, fish, milk and dairy products, processed foods, red pepper paste, soy sauce, salted fish, porridge, soup, seasoning with herbs, salt, fried foods, rice, noodles, etc. are winter or spring. We will realize how food that we have been eating has destroyed our bodies. In addition, we will understand what processed foods and additives do to our bodies. After this change, we will understand the value of this wisdom.

Ending Life after Satisfactory Living

Scott Nearing, a professor, writer, and speaker, passed away after 100 years and 28 days of living. When he realized that his time was ending, first he stopped eating solid food and drank only juice. Then, he further reduced his juice intake. At the end of his life, he only drank water and met the end of his life in this world. His last words were "Oh, good!"

Scott Nearing was a vegetarian but ate eggs and drank milk. Is it a useless idea if we contemplate that if he didn't eat cooked food, eggs, and drink milk, would he still be alive?

The average life span of a person should be between 132 and 168 years old. Many people say that we shouldn't live long or further over 80 years-old. Those people are ones who live on medication most of the time. They are people who don't realize the harm; hurting their organs by eating food without thinking about the negative and positive effects on their bodies but still worry about serious illnesses. They are not capable of dreaming about life that Scott Nearing had. If one cares about his or her organs and lives in harmony with their body, then he or she doesn't have to worry about illnesses, but can enjoy a happy life that only care and harmony would bring. When it is the end of one's life, reduce the intake of nutrition and befriend the process of the end of life like the one Scott Nearing did.

Chapter III

Diseases

Causes of Sickness

Have you ever thought about how your organs would think about the food that you eat? How you wrongly think it tastes good to you because your parents or friends eat them? Have you ever thought about the effect of the food that you eat has on your body?

We all know that if we continually eat food that harms our organs, we would get sick with diseases such as cancer, high blood pressure related illness, and dementia, but many people eat harmful food anyway with or without knowing the harmfulness of some food. We know but don't realize that our organs are an important partner for happier life. We should get permission to eat each food from our organs, "Is it fine with you if I eat this food?" We also should remind ourselves repeatedly that our organs like unprocessed and uncooked food, organic vegetables, fruits, beans, and nuts. When we treat our organs with respect and care, they will reward us with a healthier body and a happier life.

Diet

According to a survey, 62 percent of American high school students take diet pills. Elephants, rhinos, cows, and gorillas are strong and powerful, and, at the same time, they don't have any weight problems even though they eat food as much as they want. Why do young people have overweight problems? Because they were born as herbivorous animals and have been eating meat and dairy products since they were born. They have consumed cooked, instant, processed foods and have also added condiments to those foods. We should know that if we eat foods that we are made to digest, then we wouldn't have to worry about obesity, and we will be less likely have to visit the doctor's office or take medicine.

Remember

People who enjoy eating refined foods are more likely to have health problems because of malnutrition and waste piling up inside their bodies. During the processing and alteration of food, refined foods lose most of their beneficial, natural nutrients and fiber. Totally avoiding these refined foods can help us maintain a healthy weight and may reduce many health problems. So, please avoid white flour (used to make bread, pasta, pizza dough, cereal, crackers, cookies, muffin and cake), white sugar (in candy, baked goods, soda, and ice cream) and oils (in salad dressing, fried food, potato chips, baked goods and any other processed foods).

If There Was No Hypertension Drug

Generally, your blood pressure is normal if your blood pressure is less than 120/80. If your blood pressure is between 120/80 and 140/90, you are at risk of high blood pressure. If your blood pressure is higher than 140/90, your doctor will prescribe a high blood pressure medicine and recommend lifestyle modifications.

I think that many high blood pressure patients take blood pressure medicine and measure their blood pressure believing that they are in a safe range and neglect making lifestyle modifications like exercising regularly and losing weight, eating a healthy diet and reducing sodium, alcohol, caffeine, smoking, and stress. Ignoring your blood pressure is incorrect behavior because medicine puts you in danger of a heart attack. If there were no blood pressure medicines, more patients would work on lifestyle changes and save themselves.

Cancer and Protein

According to the results of various studies, protein is the switch for cancer; it can affect how the mutated cells act. In addition, according to the Journal of the National Cancer Institute, if we take protein from animal meat, it will increase the chance of developing cancer, but if we take protein from a plant then it will decrease the chance of having cancer. According to Dr. Colin Campbell, when a person takes more than 10% of his or her calories from animal protein, the chance of developing cancer increases.

Through many great studies and research, we know what cancer is and what causes it, but cancer is still the leading cause of death. Many people do not try hard enough to change their daily diet habits.

People can avoid the possibility of having cancer and the difficulties that come along with cancer treatments if they think about this while making their meals. Think about Rainbow Ssambap®.

Activated Oxygen and Antioxidants

As we get old, our body shows signs of aging such as stiff body, chronic joint pain, loss of hearing and sight due to the destructive nature of activated oxygen. Antioxidants prevent the destructive effect of activated oxygen. If we have too much activated oxygen and don't have enough antioxidants in our body, our body will slowly acidify and contract diseases such as heart problems, diabetes, asthma, fibromyalgia, emphysema, Alzheimer's, Parkinson's disease, cystic fibrosis, cancer, and aging. In order to prevent diseases, we have to supply antioxidants from outside our body since our body cannot manufacture these antioxidants. Main antioxidants are vitamin C, vitamin E, and beta-carotene.

Vitamin C is a water-soluble vitamin present in citrus fruits, juices, green peppers, cabbage, spinach, broccoli, kale, cantaloupe, kiwi, and strawberries.

Vitamin E is in nuts, seeds, vegetable, whole grains, fortified cereals, and apricots.

Beta-carotene (a precursor to vitamin A) is present in spinach, carrots, squash, broccoli, yams, tomato, cantaloupe, peaches, and grains.

Of course, Rainbow Ssambap® has these vitamins in each fruit, nut, and vegetable.

Heart Disease

Cardiovascular disease is the leading cause of death with approximately 30% of all global deaths attributed to cardiovascular disease. According to many researches and studies, a diet high in nuts, fruits, vegetables, and low in sweets, meats, dairy products and fat has been shown to reduce the risk of heart disease and death. Cardiovascular disease is treatable with initial treatment primarily focused on diet and lifestyle interventions. Rainbow Ssambap® and at least 30 minutes of exercise everyday can be considered good heart disease prevention.

Chapter IV

Food is Everything

Carnivores and Herbivores

One of the big differences between carnivores and herbivores is the length of the small intestine. Carnivores' small intestines are short and simple, but herbivores' small intestines are long and winding. Our small intestines are long and winding just like a cow's. Not only that, but there are many other indications that tell us that we are made to be herbivores, such as teeth, jaws, and acidity of the stomach. However, most people think they are omnivores and try to get their protein from eating meat or fish when we should get proteins from eating fruits, nuts, or vegetables. This mistake has been the cause of degenerative diseases, such as heart disease, cancer, and diabetes. Rich in fruit, nuts, and vegetable, Rainbow Ssambap® is one of the best foods for us herbivores.

Refined Foods

As you know, refined foods can be defined as food whose nutrient content has all been removed. These types of foods include white flour, white rice, sugar, and refined oil. When you eat refined foods, you are killing the micro flora that lives in your digestive tract. Loss of this micro flora causes constipation, creates IBS disease, and contributes to diabetes. Your inner ecosystem is slowly being poisoned to death by your addictive food cravings.

We know the harms of refined food, but we are still over-eating because many people are addicted to it. Eating refined food will artificially stimulate dopamine or the pleasure neurotransmitter in the brain; you are eating foods that cause great and happy feelings and you want more. Your heart and brain are actually being poisoned when you choose to eat refined foods.

We should free ourselves from addiction of refined foods, and it is another reason that we should eat Rainbow Ssambap®.

Refined Oil

As you know, there are two kinds of oils, unrefined and refined. Refined oil is usually cold pressed, which means the oils are mechanically extracted by a machine, which applies pressure and not heat. This leaves the high flavor and nutrient content in the oil, making them a healthier choice. Extra Virgin Olive, Avocado, Sesame, and Macadamia oils are unrefined oils.

Refined cooking oil is made by highly intensive mechanical and chemical processes to extract oil from seeds and is extracted by using heat, and a solvent, which are then bleached and deodorized. This process removes the natural nutrients from the seeds and creates a final product, which oxidizes easily. The oxidation factor makes these oils more likely to break down into cancer-causing free radicals within the body. In addition, many refined vegetable oils are also hydrogenated. This hydrogenation process further damages the fatty acids in the oils, creating trans-fatty acids, which are particularly dangerous to human health. The consumption of vegetable oils created through chemical extraction processes is linked to widespread inflammation within the body, elevated blood triglycerides, and an impaired insulin response. These oils have been linked to diabetes, cancer, and heart disease in multiple studies. Canola, Rice bran, Soya, Sunflower, and Peanut Oil are refined oils. I think the best way to get healthy fat is eating the whole seed or nut, in the state of nature. I like to eat flaxseed, which has Omega-3 fatty acids and fiber, sunflowers, and pumpkin seeds.

Dietary Vegans

Have you ever asked your organs whether they like the food that you eat? If you didn't and you eat unhealthy food, your organs will answer anyway by giving you many diseases after they've greatly suffered from your irresponsible eating. Our organs hate unnatural foods.

Our organs especially like green vegetables since they have fiber, vitamins, minerals, phytochemical, protein, calcium, and essential fatty acid, etc. Green vegetable is the best food we can eat.

If you want to get the best benefit from strictly eating vegetables, you shouldn't eat vegetables that are salted, cooked with heat, and/or mixed with refined oil and grains. Learn from animals; they can live without food that is cooked with heat, spices, and condiments.

Water

Water is our body's principal chemical component and makes up about 70 percent of our body weight. Every system in our body depends on water. For example, water flushes toxins out of vital organs, carries nutrients to our cells and provides a moist environment for our ears, nose and throat tissues. Water also increases energy and relieves fatigue since our brain is mostly water. Drinking it helps us think, focus, concentrate better, and be more alert. Water promotes weight loss, removes by-products of fat, reduces eating intake, raises your metabolism, and has zero calories. Another benefit of water is that it maintains regularity and helps relieve and prevent headaches.

Lack of water can lead to dehydration, a condition that occurs when we don't have enough water in our body to carry out normal functions. Even mild dehydration can drain our energy and make us tired.

The Institute of Medicine determined that an adequate intake (AI) for men is roughly three liters (about 13 cups) of total beverages a day. The AI for women is 2.2 liters (about 9 cups) of total beverages a day. Drink at least eight, 8-ounce glasses of fluid a day.

The Best Foods

Lemon

I think lemon is the best food that god gave to us. It has many tastes, which include sweet, acidity, salty, and bitter. Its fragrance stimulates our appetite for food. The health benefits of lemons are due to its many nourishing elements. Lemon has vitamin C, vitamin B, phosphorous, proteins, and carbohydrates. It also contains flavonoids, which are composites that contain antioxidant and cancer-fighting properties. It helps to prevent diabetes, constipation, high blood pressure, fever, indigestion and many other problems, as well as improving skin, hair, and teeth. How can so many foods do many things for us?

Tomato

Tomato is the second best food. It is sweet, juicy, and delicious. It has Vitamins A, C, K, folate and potassium. Tomatoes are naturally low in sodium, saturated fat, cholesterol, and calories. Tomatoes also provide thiamin, niacin, vitamin B6, magnesium, phosphorus, and copper, all of which are necessary for healthy body. There are many well-known health benefits: it helps protect the skin against sun damage and makes skin less sensitive to UV light damage, a leading cause of fine lines and wrinkles. It also builds strong bones; the vitamin K and calcium in tomatoes are both very good for strengthening and repairing bones. It is a natural cancer fighter. Lycopene can reduce the risk of several cancers, including prostate, cervical, mouth, pharynx, throat, esophagus, stomach, colon, rectal, prostate, and ovarian cancer. Because it contains a lot of water and fiber, it fills us up fast without adding a lot of calories or fat. There are so many that I can't talk about it all here. I eat around one hundred cherries and four regular raw tomatoes per day.

Beans

Beans are also one of the best foods and perfect replacement for meat. One of the reasons the health benefits of beans are so many is because they contain a lot of fiber and antioxidants.

According to a recent research analysis of the U.S. population and dietary practices within this population, U.S. adults would increase their intake of folate, vitamin K, calcium, magnesium, iron, and fiber if we replaced our meat and dairy intake with bean. Replacing meat and dairy with bean would also lower our total cholesterol intake. These nutritional changes, in turn, would lower our risk of several chronic diseases, including cardiovascular diseases.

When you eat dried beans, the undigested material lies around in the colon, where bacteria attacks it and starts to feed on it. In the process, many chemicals are released, which tell our liver to cut down its production of cholesterol and our blood to speed up clearing out dangerous LDL cholesterol. Moreover, fiber can actually mop up cholesterol from the intestine and whisk it out of the system. In addition, the chemicals that block formation of cancer cells are released. In fact, beans are concentrated carriers of protease inhibitors, enzymes that can counteract the activation of cancer-causing compounds in the colon.

 Other benefits of eating beans are decreasing cholesterol levels, improving diabetics' blood glucose control, reducing risk of many cancers, lowering blood pressure, regulating functions of the colon, preventing and curing constipation, preventing piles and other bowel problems.

Tofu has become a popular food among the health conscious people as great source of protein and other phytonutrients. I like to eat natural forms of beans after soaking them in water instead of being processed like tofu. I mixed the soaked bean with Rainbow Ssambap® or blend with other fruits and nuts.

Fruit

Fruits are also a wonderful food to eat. Eating fruit slows down aging and degeneration of the brain. It also reduces heart disease and blood cholesterol levels and protects us against certain types of cancers, obesity, type 2 diabetes, developing kidney stones, and helps decrease bone loss.

Fruits are naturally low in fat, sodium, and calories and none have cholesterol. Fruits are a source of many essential nutrients that are under-consumed, including potassium, dietary fiber, vitamin C, and folate (folic acid). Dietary fiber from fruits is important for proper bowel function. It helps reduce constipation and diverticulosis. It has Vitamin C, which is important for growth and repair of all body tissues, helps heal cuts and wounds, and keeps teeth and gums healthy.

Folate (folic acid) helps the body form red blood cells.

Buddah resting in my house

I hung the holy cross around his neck

He smiled

Poem- neighbors-

Phytochemical and Tomato

Phytochemicals are natural chemicals that are in plant foods. More than 25,000 phytonutrients are found in plant foods. Phytochemicals are a plant's way of protecting itself. They help shield tender buds and sprouts from predators, the elements, and pollution. These protective compounds are passed along to us when we eat plant foods. The best way to get beneficial phytochemicals that have the ability to alter body processes and protect against heart disease, cancer, hypertension, type 2 diabetes and many other chronic diseases, is eating fruits and vegetables.

A tomato has many phytochemicals such as, phytoene, phytofluene, beta-carotene, flavonoids, carotenoids, and lycopene. Lycopene is the main phytochemicals of the tomato and many health benefits of the tomato are attributed to lycopene. Studies have shown that lycopene is associated with low incidence of prostate cancer.

Rainbow Ssambap® has many phytochemicals since it has variety of fruits and vegetable. If you eat one serving of Rainbow Ssambap®, you will eat 2-3 regular tomatoes and 20-30 cherry tomatoes.

Chapter V

Nothing New, Look Novel

Be Wealthy

"Be wealthy"

It is good form of greeting. There is visible and physical wealth but then there also is an invisible and non-physical wealth. People rich in visible and physical wealth might have fancy clothes, expensive cars, and luxurious houses. They don't hesitate to spend and seem to enjoy their lives in the fullest way.

People are born with their predetermined talents for resourcefulness and the abilities of their mind (spirit). There are no two people exactly alike among so many people. Even parents and siblings are slightly different. Their personalities are different as well.

There is a whole dimension of differences ranging from a penniless homeless person to Bill Gates.

It is just like the old proverb

"You are born with your own fortune," or

"A potential tree is special even when it is a bud."

A person is born into this world with a predetermined destiny to do certain kind of jobs with how much resources and doing what kind of works to repay or fix his own karma or the original sins, to do what kind of good deeds, how to contribute to the society, and how to enlighten the spirit. People are born into the world with intents to be wealthy in spirit.

Visible and physical wealth is nothing but just a tool about how to live a life. It is useless other than to help a person become wealthy in spirit. Remember that the only thing that a person can take to the afterlife is a spirit.

Boomerang

When we look around, there are plenty of things lying about that are indecent or deserve to be criticized. Encouraged by people who gossip, anyone can criticize endlessly at these things. Criticism must be a foundation for improvement to seek fairness. A person must first be willing to self-reflect. Criticism for condemnation or slander out of spite is products of a dark heart filled with hate and jealousy. It will end up hurting the person's very own spirit (soul); however, that does not seem to bring any immediate punishment or any effect on the person. People could fall into a misconception of stress release by satisfying desires. The cause will eventually lead to the effect. Careless bullying of others for fun or manipulating others out of jealousness does return to the originator eventually in a harmful way.

Just like a boomerang.

It brings a cloud to the sunny smile on the round face that a person was born with. The cloud slowly becomes darker. Eventually it turns into a storm that rains down on a person's face.

It is the cause and effect.

It is Karma, indebtedness that must be repaid over life. Beans grow beans, not something else.

I lived a life of meditation on the mountain before. There was a pile of chestnuts under the chestnut tree in the late fall. Sitting on a rock during midday, I began peeling the chestnuts to cook chestnut rice. There were many bugs within the nuts as they were picked straight from nature. I hurt some of the bugs by mishandling the knife. I carefully cut out the parts that the bugs ate and put them over the pile of peels along with a bug. I thought I was caring for them, but then I realized that the chestnut was their home, their food, and I was the intruder, a burglar. I gasped as the realization hit me. I was doing it for the sake of feeding myself but I was pillaging the house and the food of someone else even though I was supposed to be meditating for self-reflection. Though I regretted my action, I peeled the rest of the chestnuts and ate the chestnut rice for several days afterward. All that I provided the bugs with were the peels of the chestnut and a piece of the nut that the bugs had buried.

I felt sorry.

All that I could do was hope for them to pass the winter unharmed. It was the way of the food chain so it could not have been helped. However, that act, Karma, I committed will be kept somewhere deep in my heart (spirit). It is the Karma. It is the original sin. All creatures on earth including human beings to insects are siblings born into this world to achieve paradise on earth and to enlighten the spirit (soul).

It is the law of Heaven to not only have pure actions, such as saving an endangered insect, but to also possess pure thoughts about always protecting all of nature's creatures, without exception. Further, any form of inconsideration of any kind toward anybody or anything is never to SOMETHING in the Kingdom of Heaven.

The mirrors are meant to hold images of things as they are. The mirror of the heart (spirit) is just the same. If the spirit is tied to the world of darkness, then everyday will hold misery and pain. If the spirit is always tuned in with, the world of light, then everyday will be rich and peaceful. The auspicious aura will spread to the neighbors. Good and evil will be held within the spirit as they are. The old proverb "You reap what you sow," applies.

Thinking that I am looking at

The mirror

Though I am looking at it

Poem- Mirror-

Insomnia, Depression

Excessively many people around us are suffering from insomnia. The number of people who depend on alcohol and drugs to pass the night is staggering. Without a good night's sleep, the normal life cannot continue uninterrupted. It is also a cause of the disease.

A human being is a combination of a body and a mind (spirit). Body will fatigue from physical labor. However, with a proper diet or through sleep fatigue can be cured. The energy needed for the mind (spirit) is sleep. The sleep reinvigorates the spirit and turns it active. That is why the harmony in the spirit has to be achieved to cure insomnia. We have to remove the filth from the spirit. The chaos is created from within the person himself.

We are exchange students who came to earth from the Spirit world. A task is assigned to each student. The task of life is the fear and anxiety. Students who dutifully prepared for this are confident. They know what to do. Such wisdom is earned through the habit of self-reflection. That is to do meditation of self-reflection whenever before or after the sleep. It is through the self-reflections that anxiety and fear was not visible or apparent start showing themselves.

Prejudice that only favored the one side and self-centered behavior, dark emotions that are stacked within the spirit such as hate, wrath, and the thoughts of rage, and the unstable emotion that holds all these together and the others, are the fault of oneself.

Moreover, with the continued meditation of the self-reflections the person will be rid of the flaws and start correcting them. An expert in such practice can be at ease towards even the most intolerable and unforgivable unfairness or harm as a repayment of a debt (karma or the original sins).

The person is able to raise a spirit that is strict to itself but generous to others. The person develops insight to view matters from a different perspective. That is to say that the person is returning to his once innocent and patient spirit of the baby. The innocent spirit of the baby knows where it belongs and never seeks to disrupt it from the moment of birth to death. The heaven is a place for spirits having a heart of babies. The existence of heaven (happy life where one can sleep easily) and hell (insomnia, depression) depends on the heart.

If the insomnia and depression gets unbearable to the spirit (soul) of a person then that person tries to commit suicide or may become possessed by the demon (escapee from hell). Such spirit causes most of the mental diseases. The drug, alcohol, doctors, faith, family, friends, and relatives can ease mental disease such as insomnia, depression and the others but it can never be fully cured. A game can only be won when the player plays it himself.

What would happen to the baseball game if the players sat on the stands?

An error or a failure is an experience for growth. Pain and misery is a training to enlighten the spirit and a medicine for raising the patience.

Forgiveness is for the forgiver.

> Delivered places
>
> Seated places
>
> Wherever
>
> Whenever
>
> From the heaven
>
> From the earth
>
> Wherever
>
> Whenever
>
> At sounds
>
> Poem -rain-

Meditation of Self-Reflection

To lighten your heart

For finding your true self

Do you worship at the wall?

Do you kneel and make the prayer sign with your hands?

For me,

I lie down, sit, or stand

Close or open my eyes

To ease the Spirit (heart)

To fill the Spirit

To reflect on myself

I do not read the bible of any organized religion. Abdominal breathing-based meditation of self-reflection helps improve digestion, increase concentration, and prevent or cure insomnia, cancer, and other diseases.

Life will sometimes leave a person in uncertainty, meaninglessness, and misery. Nevertheless, each of those is another opportunity for self-reflection. All suffering, such as the death of a close friend, contracting a disease, experiencing a trickery of fate, being a victim of societal ills, and receiving nothing despite giving much to provide valuable chances to self-reflect.

The most important function of self-reflection meditation is getting rid of the source of the suffering.

It is extremely effective.

The meditation of self-reflection brings back being a child of the God, to find the innocent spirit again (Matthews 18:3).

Through meditation, a person will come to ponder:

Why are human beings born?

Why do they experience pain and joy?

How do they die?

What happens in the afterlife?

A person will come to understand to live honestly.

A person comes to truly reflect on his/her past beliefs, habits, and attitudes. The gate to the vault of wisdom that a person has built for so long slowly opens. All problems, such as prejudiced minds, perverse minds, and unhealthy diets, are solved, one right after the other. The capacities for being judicious and appreciating divergent viewpoints and backgrounds are achieved.

Selflessness grows.

A road to the healing of all diseases is paved. Affection for all living things will intensify.

A person's spirituality heightens and deepens.

One learns that the wealth, status, fame, faith, body, spouse, and relatives are simply meant to be a textbook for enlightening souls (spirit). A person will realize that all the good and bad deeds to the notion of doing things but not moving into an action and everything else is carried to the afterlife.

This is a part of my experience during 100 days of camping while having two meals a day, doing meditation of self-reflection alone in the late summer to the winter of 1999.

One afternoon, while the sun is oversleeping, doing the meditation of self-reflection in the tent, overwhelmingly flooding sunlight, ecstasy after a surprise, tears raining down over a joyous heart for over an hour even at the twilight the heat on the cheeks had not cooled like a heated stone.

After that day, the meditation only deepened.

A Fly

Bashing its head on the window

Open the window

"Here you go"

Jets away

Takes a big gulp of sky

Returns to the window

Bends its knees in appreciation

Surprise!

Poem -Bow-

All by the Mind

All by the mind"
It was my motto in my youth.

I wrote it down on a paper whenever I was anxious or frustrated.

It is still my dear companion.

It means everything depends on a thought.

All by the mind.

Clinical physiologist Bob Arthur conducted a test to find out how long the conditioned response will last. He fed water mixed with saccharin and a drug to induce vomiting to a test rat. The rat was fed drugged water several times and then switched to water with just saccharin mixed into it. The result was that the rat is said to have vomited on water without the vomit-inducing drug.

Just as the test showed, everything depends on the mind (Spirit).

Any unhealthy diets can be fixed with a right mindset. Any preference for taste can be changed with a right mindset.

I never add any forms of stimulants or spices or salts to food at home. I eat and taste the nature as it is. I often suffered from indigestion since childhood but with the rigorous training exercise and meals provided by the army, which included simple rice and soups, my condition had improved a bit. After recovering from colitis in 6 months and returning to duty, I vowed to improve my diet. I refused to use any drugs (i.e., medicine). I did not consume any soups, stews, pickles, or any food that was salty or stimulants. I avoided coffee, tea, soft drinks, and any refreshments with caffeine, sugar, and other additives. I quit the cigarettes too. I avoided as many artificial foods as possible. Then within 6 months, I was able to regain my perfect health. As of today, I am 72 years old but I continue to enjoy my good health without any aid from drugs or health supplements (i.e., daily diet and exercise). All of my health indicators are normal.

The taste of food is influenced by dietary habits. If people who enjoyed a salty and strong taste were to somehow change their diets into pure and clean foods, void of substance, such as, mayonnaise, salt, and spicier, after time, their complete sense of taste would dramatically change. These same individuals would soon be overwhelmed by salty and spicy foods to the point of rejecting them.

Digestive systems that cannot cope with salty and spicy foods, which only satisfy the mouth, will lead to an illness. Though it may sound unbelievable, do not forget that each organ has its own consciousness (Soul). Even though a taste may be extremely pleasant to tongue and mouth, it may simultaneously be very injurious to the digestive system. In other words, the digestive system as an organ with its own mind, feels betrayed by the indulgences of the body or "master," to the point of not being able to serve it any longer [giving up on the master in the form of a disease (Karma) which is sometimes deadly].

There is no such thing as an unfixable habit.

Children will often mimic the habits of their parents. Is it right then, to allow the children to develop a habit of depending on the doctors in search of medicines because of their bad diets consisting of hamburgers, chili, and tacos, which they learned from their parents?

It is time for the young fathers and mothers to think about what it means to parent responsibly.

It is time to take the initiative for the future well-being of the children and the parents.

All problems and bad habits are a product of uncontrolled greed and desires. No one can deceive oneself or do two things at once. If a person thinks of evil then that person will be led to Hell. If a person thinks of good then that person's Spirit will be led to heaven. Bad diets of salty and spicy foods may suit the mouth but the digestive systems will suffer.

A stupidity is the source of all diseases.

Such a phenomenon of countless results originating from a single thought is called "A single notion, with three thousand outcomes."

Not being obsessed with wealth, fame, or status and maintaining a good diet, Spirit, life, and living every moment to its fullest without regret, is called "Carpe diem."

You who memorizes and remembers, a hundred times a day, the tares' ideas of, "All by The mind,"

"A single notion, there thousand outcomes," and "carpe diem," will lead a Heavenly life today and tomorrow.

To the Field
To the Mountains
To the Ocean
Went everywhere

Things like these
Things like those
Things like other

Sights to see
Sounds to hear
Neither seen or heard

However
Be as true self
Naturally
Got along well

The heaven clock
With a smile
Opens the road for Earth things
Closed the road for Earth things

Poem —The Heaven Clock-

A Body and a Spirit

According to science, the cerebral cortex is where the reasoning, memorization, and dreams happen. Science argues that since all human feelings and sensations are the product of the brain's activity, should the brain cease to function then that will be the end of everything.

If that is so, then how come, even though every sensory organ should be working properly, that no one can hear or smell anything while asleep?

This is the mystery that medical science cannot figure out.

Sleep rests the body but the reason that a body cannot receive any information while asleep is because the spirit (heart) is away from body to receive energies from the heaven. The spirit is linked to the body via spirit-body line (ref: Death) so that the spirit (heart) may return to the body whenever needed. Spirit is the true entity that wanders between two realms of this world and the Spirit world. The brain and the five senses are mere servants that do the biddings of the spirit (heart). Therefore, we must try to understand the true nature of our spirit (mind).

Our mind is occupied by both the good and evil.
Therefore, we have to learn to control our wrath,
jealousy, spite, stubbornness, and obsession and be
benevolent and considerate of the others. No one
can deceive oneself. People lie to the others for
manipulation so the liars may benefit themselves or to
avoid the punishment. Such actions and thoughts are
undoubtedly recorded into a mind (spirit).

Karma (original sins) has to be repaid.

When we learn to be content with our own life and
free of desires to amass wealth or fame, then we can
find the true value of life. We can lead a fair life that
emerges from our spirit (heart) and through our five
senses.

We learn that all of us are of the God's image and
parts of him. We then understand the power of
creation and a freedom of choice. Through the
sensible creativity by the righteous choice, we expand
and deepen our innocence to become one with the
God. Reaching closer to the perfection. (Christ,
Buddha).

When sky was low and the malicious wind was

brutally chilly

I suddenly encountered one on the path

covered with the dead vegetation

One tiny flower

Smiling brightly

"Straigten your body, please!"

Whipped my shoulder with a bamboo stick

Poem -The Bamboo Stick of an Awakening

*A Bamboo stick that master uses to awaken monks who dozed off while meditating.

For the humanity, for the nature

It is said that the God was happy for a while after the sky and the earth was created as all creatures lived along fine with each other without any trouble. However, if there was one thing that had bothered him then it was a creature called human that was crafty and a little too clever for its own good. He was worried that humans might unbalance the world so while everyone was a sleep, he changed the human's digestive system to be compatible with the vegetables. After that event, there were not any problems up to the agriculture era. Then something called the Industrial Revolution started from Britain fuming the dark smokes had bothered the God. Floating man made birds up in the sky, creating various man killing machines, invoking a massive bloodshed.

The God is said to have been unable to breath.

The sunlight sparkles the spring sea

Thousands of anchovies wearing the peaked hat
join the exciting party.

Packed seagulls rise

Anchovies fall

Crashing the forehead against the rock
The boiling wave

A tightly sealed lip
The horizon

Poem-The Spring Sea:
The current Middle East event-

Now driven by the greed of wealth, they have invented unimaginable chemical fertilizers to food additives, growth hormone, antibiotic, and pesticides to cause an indirect murder and damage to the soil. However, the people suffer from the diseases and early deaths caused by the unhealthy consumption of meats and though there are even more countless people dying from the starvation around the world, 1/3 of the world's grain are fed to the livestock instead of to the people (US feeds 70% of the national grain supply to the livestock). In addition, refusing to stop there, livestock such as pig, chicken and cattle are put into a horrible condition of living and forced into growth acceleration so that their meat can be produced in larger quantity and in better quality.

God who was unable to see it continue any further gave a call. It is time to end it he said.

Even after all the cautions and advices, this is the fourth time (according to the elder of the Hopi Indians, this is the peak of the fourth humanity) that this has happened and though it pains him to do it, the God says that there are no alternatives to stop the humanity's over-consumption.

In the fifth humanity, people will have pure eyes as the deer do and will be unable to stand so that they can only feed on vegetation.
There shall be no more wars, or conflicts between religions, unnecessary educations, or polluting of science.

There shall be a paradise on earth where conflicts, obsession, over-consumption, wrath, arrogance, or suicide and other such economic and social problems will be rid of. Just as all animals that live past 6~7 times the growth period, humans will live 132~168 years. There shall be no more need for any of the doctors and hospitals. Therefore, few of those past their 100 years today will be treated as young.

Looking at the dictionary
Nothing is missing

As the autumn deepens
Grabbing the rake
Holding the sack

Saying that he will scoop the moon up from
the pond

Saying that he will capture the wave from
the shore

Poem -Futility:
Including the poem writing-

Two Sides of a Coin

Try to look back to the day before sleeping.

If it was a good day then you will have a good night sleep and a dream.

If it was a bad day then you will not be able to comfortably rest at all. You may suffer from the nightmares.

The day-to-day life of this world is the day-to-day life of the Spirit world. Just as the today's sun will rise again tomorrow, the life of this world is linked to the Spirit world.

In religions, a day that followed its doctrine will be rewarded with an invitation to the heavenly tomorrow.

In addition, a day that contradicted its doctrine will receive a punishment from hell.

The purity of the spirit of a person will determine the outcome of his afterlife that is either happy or hellish, just like the fate of the farmer is decided by his crop.

One decides the life of the afterlife. It is related to the size of the spiritual window of the person.

Those who try to forcefully enter the world of happiness that they do not deserve will find themselves unbearable and blinded by its brightness, and they must find their way back to the place where they should belong. Those who do not farm dutifully will find themselves plunging into the deeper depths of the underworld, to the world of hell. That is the unforgiving law of the heaven.

There is no such thing as a divine punishment in this world or in the Spirit world. One reaps what one sows. That is the only divine law that the God has given along with a freedom of choice and creation. Just like how the system of the sentence or ignominy works, the disease is a result of the foul deeds done against the organs. Disease, anxiety, or hell cannot approach the ones with a heart of an innocent child.

The window of the spirit is the purity, clarity, and light of the heart (spirit). All of the creatures that live, be they insignificant as insects, are siblings born into this world for the sake of enlightening the spirit. We have to live with a kind spirit and honesty and conform to the nature.

To cast a fishing rod without a hook
trying to catch the moon
Careful of the busy ants
Careful of the root of a tree
a caring heart.

They, who try to serve themselves with a visible, skin
deep, earthly knowledge instead of trying to open
their spiritual window, will lose their honesty in heart.
Their heart (spirit) will be directed to the hell.

A droplet of water creates an ocean.

This world and the Spirit world are not separate.
They are two parts of a bigger world.
Look at the both sides of the coin.
They are inseparable.
The life of this world and the life of the Spirit world is a
single life in an even bigger world.
A life like two sides of a coin.

> Deep in the mountain
> A small thatched hut
> A small lamp
>
> A big round moon
> A yard full of light
>
> A twosome
> A world full of love
>
> Poem -Twosome-

You Are An Artist

You are an artist.

You were born an artist.

God gave us the freedom of choice and creation.

We can draw whatever our hearts desire.

Since you have the hand of God.

Who creates beauty and dreams.

The painting is a product of creativity.

It is a process of drawing out a hidden ability.

It is pure water that our hearts (spirit) possess.

The flashing inspiration is the act of flushing out

pure spring water.

The expressions of children are very bright.

They are innocent, just like nature.

Children draw pictures very simply.

Their drawing is always simple, whether they are

illustrating their mother or their father.

It is because their hearts are pure and clean.

Let us all return to our childhood.

Let us enjoy the freedom of choice and creation to its fullest.

An example of the freedom of choice would be to choose salad for dinner. Freedom of creation happens when that same individual actually prepared the salad.

Parents, companions, friends, religions, jobs, etc., are the results of choices made.

God does not intervene into the lives of others; therefore, all outcomes are the products of individual choices made in our daily lives.

All people must bear the responsibility of their actions.

It is the absolute God-made law of Heaven.

If God intervened in everyone's daily lives, the world would have been a paradise a long time ago.

Now prepare to do some painting.

Get some paints, a canvas, and a brush.

Use acrylic for paint.

It is a good paint that the older masters of art

would have liked to use.

Acrylic is almost odorless, and it dries quickly.

You can keep reusing the brush left in water.

Have the frames ready, too.

The last autumn has been very memorable.

I strolled the forest while holding His hand.

There is a tree with many ripe fruits.

The birds helped themselves to persimmons,

which made them sing.

Autumn leaves smile colorfully.

The Cosmos dances to and fro.

He, the mountains, and everyone smiles.

The paradise that I once dreamed of, opens slowly.

You are the creator of the paradise on the canvas.

The pure heart stands in front of the canvas.

You are the angel, the sage.

First draw six overlapping circles.

These will be the head, body, arms, and legs.

Draw the smile in the top circle.

The smile binds everything together, and you

stand next to it.

The two smiling beings are happy.

Then paint the mountain, persimmon tree,

flowers, and the birds.

When the sun smiles, everyone smiles back.

Then dress everyone in their own clothes, and colors.

The black dress is for the persimmon tree, the blue

is for the persimmons, and because you are the

creator, the choices are all yours to make.

Erasing or changing anything is up to you as well.

Frame the painting.

It is completed whether or not you are satisfied

with the piece.

Creation has thousands of expressions.

Enjoy the fact that you have finished.

You will be focused upon your creation for a little while.

It will look pretty no matter what anyone says about it.

It is a pair of glasses for your sight.

If someone criticizes your painting, you will be upset.

Then, all of a sudden, at a later time, you will understand.

The critic was being objectively honest.

It was because he perceived your creation from another point of view.

You were too consumed with anger, and it clouded your judgment.

It was a time when you were too defensive.

Such a phenomenon is caused by emotion overriding reason.

It is difficult to make a logical decision.

It is a time in which you do not want to listen to any differing opinions, or to feel humiliated.

In your mind, there are many hidden obsessions and feelings of wrath.

You must burn the coals of wrath and obsessions, one by one.

That is why you must paint.

Do not forget to smile, no matter who tries to criticize or hurt you.

That is the only way for you to give your smiles to others.

That is the only way to become a happy artist.

And you help make the world more bright and clear.

You, who properly handles God's gift of,

"The Freedom of Choice and Creation".

Birds do not leave holes in the sky

They embrace the wind to lift from the earth

Poem **Airplane**

Sleeping leaf

All leaves

Suckle milk

'Till the noontime

Poem **Dew**

www.ingramcontent.com/pod-product-compliance
Lightning Source LLC
Chambersburg PA
CBHW060339290526
45793CB00003B/668